FREEDOM FROM SLEEP DISORDER

DIVINE MEDICINE THAT WORKS

BY
IHEKE WILLIAMS

COPYRIGHT © 2019, IHEKE WILLIAMS

All rights reserved under International Copyright Law. Contents and/or cover may not be reproduced in whole or in part in any form without the express written permission of Iheke Williams.

Unless otherwise indicated, all scripture quotations are taken from the King James Version of the Bible. A key for other Bible versions used;

NKJV	New King James Version
AMP	The Amplified Bible
TANT	The New Amplified Bible
TLB -	The Living Bible
CEV -	Contemporary English Version
NASB	New American Standard Version
GW -	God's Word version
ESV -	English Standard Version
NET -	New English Translation
ISV -	International Standard Version
NIV -	New International Version
MSG -	The Message Translation

DEDICATION

This Book is dedicated to Almighty God and to our Lord Jesus Christ.

TABLE OF CONTENT

FREEDOM FROM SLEEP DISORDER
COPYRIGHT © 2019, IHEKE WILLIAMS
DEDICATION
TABLE OF CONTENT
WHAT IS SLEEP DISORDER?
WHAT IS GOD'S SOLUTION?
INSTRUCTION 1
INSTRUCTION 2
AFFIRMATION DAY 1
AFFIRMATION DAY 2
AFFIRMATION DAY 3
AFFIRMATION DAY 4
AFFIRMATION DAY 5
AFFIRMATION DAY 6
AFFIRMATION DAY 7
AFFIRMATION DAY 8
AFFIRMATION DAY 9
AFFIRMATION DAY 10
AFFIRMATION DAY 11
AFFIRMATION DAY 12
AFFIRMATION DAY 13
AFFIRMATION DAY 14
AFFIRMATION DAY 15
AFFIRMATION DAY 16
AFFIRMATION DAY 17
AFFIRMATION DAY 18
AFFIRMATION DAY 19
AFFIRMATION DAY 20
AFFIRMATION DAY 21
AFFIRMATION DAY 22
AFFIRMATION DAY 23
AFFIRMATION DAY 24
AFFIRMATION DAY 25
AFFIRMATION DAY 26
AFFIRMATION DAY 27
AFFIRMATION DAY 28
AFFIRMATION DAY 29
AFFIRMATION DAY 30
AFFIRMATION DAY 31
SUMMARY
PRAYER FOR SALVATION
OTHER INFORMATION
ABOUT THE AUTHOR

WHAT IS SLEEP DISORDER?

Sleep disorders are changes in the way that you sleep.

A sleep disorder can affect your overall health, safety and quality of life. Sleep deprivation can affect your ability to drive safely and increase your risk of other health problems.

Some of the signs and symptoms of sleep disorders include excessive daytime sleepiness, irregular breathing or increased movement during sleep, and difficulty falling asleep.

There are many different types of sleep disorders. They're often grouped into categories that explain why they happen or how they affect you. Sleep disorders can also be grouped according to behaviors, problems with your natural sleep-wake cycles, breathing problems, difficulty sleeping or how sleepy you feel during the day.

Source: Mayo Clinic Health Centre

WHAT IS GOD'S SOLUTION

"But He was wounded for our transgressions, he was bruised for our iniquities: the chastisement of our peace was upon Him; and with His stripes we are healed – Isaiah 53:5 (KJV)

"...By His wounds ye have been healed" –
1 Peter 2:24 (KJV)

The phrase "...ye **HAVE BEEN HEALED**" is in the past tense, it means JESUS CHRIST has ALREADY HEALED you from sleeping disorder, years ago.

You have NO business with sleeping disorders.

Your sleep has been restored a long time ago. So start sleeping well. Halleluyah!! Thanks be to God the Almighty.

For the next 31 days and Forever, you will affirm this blessing that Our Lord Jesus Christ has given to you and you will you live in perfect health FOREVER!.

INSTRUCTIONS

That if thou shalt <u>confess w</u>... Lord Jesus, and shalt <u>believe in</u>... God hath raised him from the dea... be saved. – Romans 10:9

We having the same <u>spirit of faith</u>, accordi... it is written, I believed, and therefore have... spoken; <u>we also believe, and therefore speak</u>; – 2 Corinthians 4:13

There has to be a connection with what you say/affirm with your mouth and what you have in your heart or what you believe with your heart.

Consequently, for the affirmations to be effective, you will have to meditate on the scripture (1 Peter 2:24) for 5 minutes, in your heart, before you affirm it with your mouth.

Don't say anything to the contrary during the period of affirmations.

INSTRUCTION 2

'For our light affliction, which is but for a moment, worketh for us a far more exceeding and eternal weight of glory;

<u>While we look not at the things which are seen</u>, but at the things which <u>are not seen</u>: for the things which are seen are temporal; but <u>the things which are not seen are eternal</u>. –
2 Corinthians 4:17-18 (KJV)

For the duration of the affirmations, do not touch any part of your body that might have been affected by this sickness. If it is possible, don't look at it.

The word of God (1 Peter 2:24) in your heart will <u>not</u> be effective when you keep recognizing the presence of a sickness because doubt will begin to develop in your heart and the word doesn't work in the presence of doubts/unbelief.

Follow these instructions, **BE CONSISTENT** and your affirmations will be very effective.

DAY 1
AFFIRMATION

Meditate on 1 Peter 2:24B in your heart for 5 minutes

"..By His stripes ye have been healed"

Now affirm the Blessing

"I HAVE BEEN HEALED THEREFORE, I AFFIRM THAT I AM FREE FROM ALL FORMS OF SICKNESS FOREVER!"

DAY 2
AFFIRMATION

Meditate on 1 Peter 2:24B in your heart for 5 minutes

"..By His stripes ye have been healed"

Now affirm the Blessing

"I HAVE BEEN HEALED THEREFORE, I AFFIRM THAT I DO NOT HAVE SLEEP DISORDER!"

DAY 3
AFFIRMATION

Meditate on 1 Peter 2:24B in your heart for 5 minutes

"..By His stripes ye have been healed"

Now affirm the Blessing

"I HAVE BEEN HEALED THEREFORE, I AFFIRM THAT MY SLEEP IS ACTIVE AND STRONG FOREVER!!"

DAY 4
AFFIRMATION

Meditate on 1 Peter 2:24B in your heart for 5 minutes

"..By His stripes ye have been healed"

Now affirm the Blessing

"I HAVE BEEN HEALED THEREFORE, I AFFIRM THAT I AM FREE FROM SLEEP DISORDER FOREVER!"

DAY 5
AFFIRMATION

Meditate on 1 Peter 2:24B in your heart for 5 minutes

"..By His stripes ye have been healed"

Now affirm the Blessing

"I HAVE BEEN HEALED THEREFORE, I AFFIRM THAT I HAVE GOOD SLEEP!!"

DAY 6
AFFIRMATION

Meditate on 1 Peter 2:24B in your heart for 5 minutes

"..**By His stripes ye have been healed**"

Now affirm the Blessing

"I HAVE BEEN HEALED THEREFORE, I AFFIRM THAT MY SLEEP IS ACTIVE AND STRONG FOREVER!!"

DAY 7
AFFIRMATION

Meditate on 1 Peter 2:24B in your heart for 5 minutes

"..By His stripes ye have been healed"

Now affirm the Blessing

"I HAVE BEEN HEALED THEREFORE, I AFFIRM THAT I DO NOT HAVE SLEEP DISORDER!"

DAY 8
AFFIRMATION

Meditate on 1 Peter 2:24B in your heart for 5 minutes

"..By His stripes ye have been healed"

Now affirm the Blessing

"I HAVE BEEN HEALED THEREFORE, I AFFIRM THAT MY SLEEP IS ACTIVE AND STRONG FOREVER!!"

DAY 9
AFFIRMATION

Meditate on 1 Peter 2:24B in your heart for 5 minutes

"..By His stripes ye have been healed"

Now affirm the Blessing

"I HAVE BEEN HEALED THEREFORE, I AFFIRM THAT I DO NOT HAVE SLEEP DISORDER!"

DAY 10
AFFIRMATION

Meditate on 1 Peter 2:24B in your heart for 5 minutes

"..By His stripes ye have been healed"

Now affirm the Blessing

"I HAVE BEEN HEALED THEREFORE, I AFFIRM THAT I HAVE GOOD SLEEP!!"

DAY 11
AFFIRMATION

Meditate on 1 Peter 2:24B in your heart for 5 minutes

"..By His stripes ye have been healed"

Now affirm the Blessing

"I HAVE BEEN HEALED THEREFORE, I AFFIRM THAT I AM FREE FROM SLEEP DISORDER FOREVER!"

DAY 12
AFFIRMATION

Meditate on 1 Peter 2:24B in your heart for 5 minutes

"..By His stripes ye have been healed"

Now affirm the Blessing

"I HAVE BEEN HEALED THEREFORE, I AFFIRM THAT I DO NOT HAVE SLEEP DISORDER!"

DAY 13
AFFIRMATION

Meditate on 1 Peter 2:24B in your heart for 5 minutes

"..By His stripes ye have been healed"

Now affirm the Blessing

"I HAVE BEEN HEALED THEREFORE, I AFFIRM THAT MY SLEEP IS ACTIVE AND STRONG FOREVER!!"

DAY 14
AFFIRMATION

Meditate on 1 Peter 2:24B in your heart for 5 minutes

"..By His stripes ye have been healed"

Now affirm the Blessing

"I HAVE BEEN HEALED THEREFORE, I AFFIRM THAT I AM FREE FROM SLEEP DISORDER FOREVER!"

DAY 15
AFFIRMATION

Meditate on 1 Peter 2:24B in your heart for 5 minutes

"..By His stripes ye have been healed"

Now affirm the Blessing

"I HAVE BEEN HEALED THEREFORE, I AFFIRM THAT I HAVE GOOD SLEEP!!"

DAY 16
AFFIRMATION

Meditate on 1 Peter 2:24B in your heart for 5 minutes

"..By His stripes ye have been healed"

Now affirm the Blessing

"I HAVE BEEN HEALED THEREFORE, I AFFIRM THAT MY SLEEP IS ACTIVE AND STRONG FOREVER!!"

DAY 17
AFFIRMATION

Meditate on 1 Peter 2:24B in your heart for 5 minutes

"..By His stripes ye have been healed"

Now affirm the Blessing

"I HAVE BEEN HEALED THEREFORE, I AFFIRM THAT I DO NOT HAVE SLEEP DISORDER!"

DAY 18
AFFIRMATION

Meditate on 1 Peter 2:24B in your heart for 5 minutes

"..By His stripes ye have been healed"

Now affirm the Blessing

"I HAVE BEEN HEALED THEREFORE, I AFFIRM THAT MY SLEEP IS ACTIVE AND STRONG FOREVER!!"

DAY 19
AFFIRMATION

Meditate on 1 Peter 2:24B in your heart for 5 minutes

"..By His stripes ye have been healed"

Now affirm the Blessing

"I HAVE BEEN HEALED THEREFORE, I AFFIRM THAT I AM FREE FROM SLEEP DISORDER FOREVER!"

DAY 20
AFFIRMATION

Meditate on 1 Peter 2:24B in your heart for 5 minutes

"..By His stripes ye have been healed"

Now affirm the Blessing

"I HAVE BEEN HEALED THEREFORE, I AFFIRM THAT I HAVE GOOD SLEEP!!"

DAY 21
AFFIRMATION

Meditate on 1 Peter 2:24B in your heart for 5 minutes

"..By His stripes ye have been healed"

Now affirm the Blessing

"I HAVE BEEN HEALED THEREFORE, I AFFIRM THAT I DO NOT HAVE SLEEP DISORDER!"

DAY 22
AFFIRMATION

Meditate on 1 Peter 2:24B in your heart for 5 minutes

"..By His stripes ye have been healed"

Now affirm the Blessing

"I HAVE BEEN HEALED THEREFORE, I AFFIRM THAT I AM FREE FROM SLEEP SICKNESS FOREVER!"

DAY 23
AFFIRMATION

Meditate on 1 Peter 2:24B in your heart for 5 minutes

"..By His stripes ye have been healed"

Now affirm the Blessing

"I HAVE BEEN HEALED THEREFORE, I AFFIRM THAT MY SLEEP IS ACTIVE AND STRONG FOREVER!!"

DAY 24
AFFIRMATION

Meditate on 1 Peter 2:24B in your heart for 5 minutes

"..By His stripes ye have been healed"

Now affirm the Blessing

"I HAVE BEEN HEALED THEREFORE, I AFFIRM THAT I AM FREE FROM SLEEP DISORDER FOREVER!"

DAY 25
AFFIRMATION

Meditate on 1 Peter 2:24B in your heart for 5 minutes

"..By His stripes ye have been healed"

Now affirm the Blessing

"I HAVE BEEN HEALED THEREFORE, I AFFIRM THAT I HAVE GOOD SLEEP!!"

DAY 26
AFFIRMATION

Meditate on 1 Peter 2:24B in your heart for 5 minutes

"..By His stripes ye have been healed"

Now affirm the Blessing

"I HAVE BEEN HEALED THEREFORE, I AFFIRM THAT MY SLEEP IS ACTIVE AND STRONG FOREVER!!"

DAY 27
AFFIRMATION

Meditate on 1 Peter 2:24B in your heart for 5 minutes

"..By His stripes ye have been healed"

Now affirm the Blessing

"I HAVE BEEN HEALED THEREFORE, I AFFIRM THAT I DO NOT HAVE SLEEP DISORDER!"

DAY 28
AFFIRMATION

Meditate on 1 Peter 2:24B in your heart for 5 minutes

"..By His stripes ye have been healed"

Now affirm the Blessing

"I HAVE BEEN HEALED THEREFORE, I AFFIRM THAT MY SLEEP IS ACTIVE AND STRONG FOREVER!!"

DAY 29
AFFIRMATION

Meditate on 1 Peter 2:24B in your heart for 5 minutes

"..By His stripes ye have been healed"

Now affirm the Blessing

"I HAVE BEEN HEALED THEREFORE, I AFFIRM THAT I DO NOT HAVE SLEEP DISORDER!"

DAY 30
AFFIRMATION

Meditate on 1 Peter 2:24B in your heart for 5 minutes

"..By His stripes ye have been healed"

Now affirm the Blessing

"I HAVE BEEN HEALED THEREFORE, I AFFIRM THAT I HAVE
GOOD SLEEP!!"

DAY 31
AFFIRMATION

Meditate on 1 Peter 2:24B in your heart for 5 minutes

"..By His stripes ye have been healed"

Now affirm the Blessing

"I HAVE BEEN HEALED THEREFORE, I AFFIRM THAT I AM FREE FROM SLEEP DISORDER FOREVER!"

"..by His stripes ye HAVE BEEN HEALED"- 1 PETER 2:24

Jesus Christ has paid the price for your peace. Don't let Satan deceive you that you are sick.

Don't let Satan put you in bondage any longer.

Your body has been healed already. You have NO business with sickness.

You are ACTIVE AND STRONG FOREVER!

You are **FREE FOREVER**!

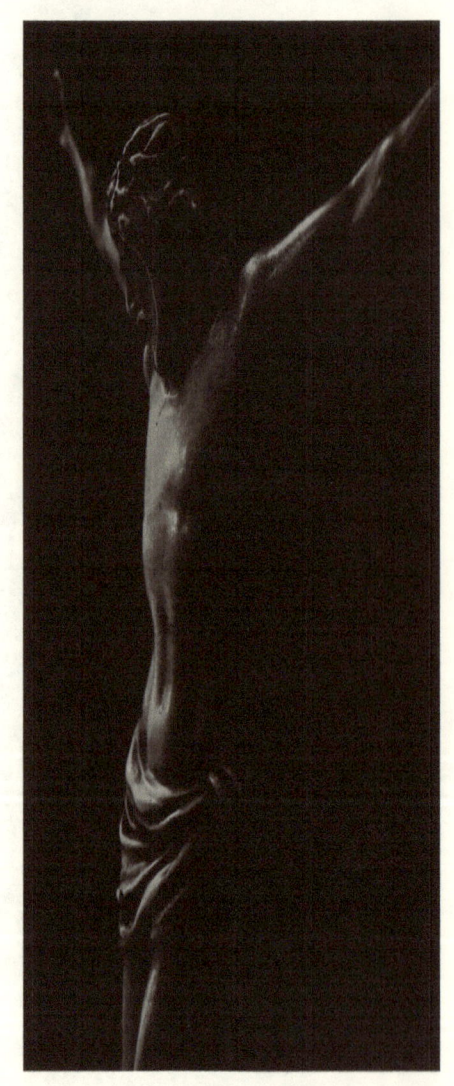

PRAYER FOR SALVATION

We believe that you have been blessed and that you want to receive eternal life that God has made available to everyone who believes in his love and his grace which He expressed lavishly through His Son Jesus Christ.

"For God so loved the world, that He gave his only begotten Son, that whosoever <u>believeth</u> in him should not perish, but <u>have everlasting life.</u>" - John 3:16

Say this prayer to God and believe it with your heart

"Father, I believe that you gave me your only Son to die for my sin. I believe you raised Him from the dead. I declare that your son, Jesus Christ is the Lord of my life. I receive eternal life and I receive the Holy Spirit. I am saved forever.in Jesus name. I am so Happy that today and forever, I am your child. Amen ".

Congratulations, you are now a child of God Halleluyah!! – John 1:12

OTHER INFORMATION

Please share your testimonies via the following handles;

ihekewilliams@gmail.com
+2348061530541

Other Books written by the author includes

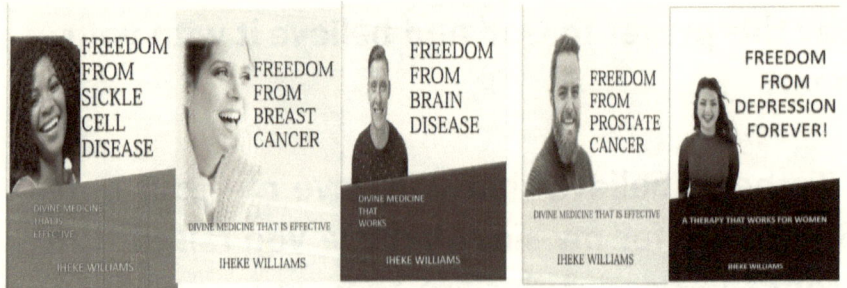

Visit us on Amazon by clicking on the link below;

https://www.amazon.com/Iheke-w.-Okpara/e/B01KFYO1PU/ref=ntt_dp_epwbk_0

ABOUT THE AUTHOR

Iheke Williams is a firm follower and disciple of the Lord Jesus Christ. He is a passionate minister of the grace of our Lord and savior Jesus Christ and has brought the reality of the divine life of Christ into the lives of so many.

Iheke Williams has a calling to communicate the gospel of Christ with simplicity and to show the world how to activate the eternal life of God that is in us already which includes Divine health, Divine righteousness, Divine security and Divine prosperity.

As you read this book and other books written by Iheke Williams you will literally begin to function and manifest the life of God that is already inside you to the glory of God the Father who is the author of all grace and mercy. Amen.

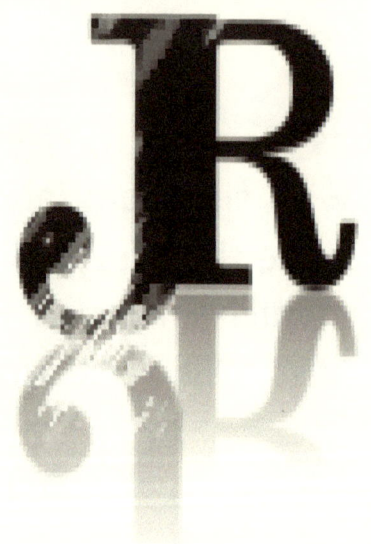

"..by His stripes ye
<u>HAVE BEEN HEALED</u>"-
1 PETER 2:24

YOU
ARE
FREE
FOREVER!!

www.ingramcontent.com/pod-product-compliance
Lightning Source LLC
Chambersburg PA
CBHW021939170526
45157CB00005B/2355